WHAT MEDICINE CAN DO FOR LAW

By BENJAMIN N. CARDOZO

CHIEF JUSTICE, COURT OF APPEALS
STATE OF NEW YORK

The Anniversary Discourse
delivered before
The New York Academy of Medicine
November 1, 1928

THE LAWBOOK EXCHANGE, LTD.
Clark, New Jersey

ISBN 978-1-58477-669-7

Lawbook Exchange edition 2005, 2014

The quality of this reprint is equivalent to the quality of the original work.

THE LAWBOOK EXCHANGE, LTD.
33 Terminal Avenue
Clark, New Jersey 07066-1321

*Please see our website for a selection of our other publications
and fine facsimile reprints of classic works of legal history:*
www.lawbookexchange.com

Library of Congress Cataloging-in-Publication Data

Cardozo, Benjamin N. (Benjamin Nathan), 1870-1938.
  What medicine can do for law / Benjamin N. Cardozo.
    p. cm.
  Originally published: New York, London : Harper & Brothers, 1930.
  ISBN 1-58477-669-2 (alk. paper)
  1. Medical jurisprudence--United States. I. Title.
KF3821.C373 2006
344.7304'1--dc22   2005005597

Printed in the United States of America on acid-free paper

WHAT MEDICINE CAN DO FOR LAW

By BENJAMIN N. CARDOZO

CHIEF JUSTICE, COURT OF APPEALS
STATE OF NEW YORK

*The Anniversary Discourse
delivered before
The New York Academy of Medicine
November 1, 1928*

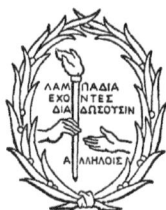

NEW YORK AND LONDON
Harper & Brothers Publishers
1930

What Medicine Can Do for Law

What Medicine Can Do for Law

THERE are those who say that the earliest physician was the priest, just as the earliest judge was the ruler who uttered the divine command and was king and priest combined. Modern scholarship warns us to swallow with a grain of salt these sweeping generalities, yet they have at least a core of truth. Our professions — yours and mine — medicine and law — have divided with the years, yet they were not far apart at the beginning. There hovered over each the nimbus of a tutelage that was supernatural, if not divine. To this day each retains for the other a trace of the thaumaturgic quality distinctive of its origin. The physician is still the wonder-worker, the soothsayer, to whose reading of the entrails we resort when hard beset. We may scoff at him in health, but we send for him in pain. The judge, if you fall into his clutches, is still the Themis of the Greeks, announcing mystic dooms. You may not understand his words, but their effects you can be made to feel. Each of us is thus a man of mystery to the other, a power to be propitiated in proportion to the element within it that is mystic or unknown. "Speak not ill of a great enemy," says Selden in his *Table-Talk* — and Selden, you must know, was one of the ancient sages of our law,— "speak not ill of a great enemy, but rather give him good words that he may use you the better if you chance to fall into his hands. The Spaniard did this when he was dying; his confessor told him, to work him to repentance, how the Devil tormented the wicked that went to hell; the Spaniard replying called the Devil my Lord; I hope my Lord the Devil is not so cruel. His confessor reproved him; excuse me for calling him so, says the Don, I know not into what hands I may fall, and if I happen into his, I hope he will use me the better for giving him good words." So with judges and doctors and devils it is all one, at least in hours of extremity.

One of these hours of extremity is at hand, the hour for the delivery of an anniversary address. The president of your Academy, moved I know not by what impulse — perhaps by some such faint foreboding as shaped the words of the Don in addressing his confessor — has turned with fair and soft speech to one without the mystic guild and has called upon a judge to preach the lesson of the hour. This is extraordinary enough, yet still more extraordinary is the fact that the judge has responded to the summons. In thus responding he has not been beguiled into the vain belief that any message he has to offer is worthy of your patience. He disclaims even a faint foreboding that there is need to propitiate your favor as against some future hour when he may be driven to seek your ministrations in default of other aid. Nothing is there on his side except a gesture of mere friendliness, the friendliness that is due between groups united in a common quest, the quest for the rule of order, the rule of health and of disease, to which for individuals as for society we give the name of law.

Indeed, the more I think it over, the more I feel the closeness of the tie that binds our guilds together. In all this there is nothing strange. I was reading the other day a very interesting document, a report to the overseers of Harvard University by the president of the university, Dr. A. Lawrence Lowell. He speaks of a new educational concept, the concept, as he calls it, of the continuity of knowledge. The idea is taking root that the subdivisions of science, like those of time itself, have been treated too often as absolute and genuine — that there is need to recognize them more fully as mere figments of the brain, mere labor-saving devices, helps to thinking, but like other helps to thinking, misleading if their origin is neglected or forgotten. Thus it is that the physicist is learning from the chemist, the zoologist from the botanist, the economist from the statesman and the student of social science, the physician from the psychologist, and so on interchangeably and indefinitely. "The sharp severance," we are told, "is giving way, and we perceive that all subjects pass imperceptibly into others previously distinct." Something of this same concept of the continuity of knowledge is making its way into the law. In my own court at a recent session we had one case where a wise decision called for the wisdom of a chemist; another for that of one skilled in the science of mechanics; another for that of the student of biology and medicine; and so on through the list. I do not say we were able to supply this fund of wisdom out of the resources of our knowledge, yet in theory, at least, the litigants before us were entitled to expect it, and our efficiency as judges would be so much the greater, the quality of the output so much

the sounder and richer, in proportion to our
ability to make the theory one with fact. More
and more we lawyers are awaking to a perception
of the truth that what divides and distracts us
in the solution of a legal problem is not so much
uncertainty about the law as uncertainty about
the facts — the facts which generate the law.
Let the facts be known as they are, and the law
will sprout from the seed and turn its branches
toward the light. We make our blunders from
time to time as rumor has it that you make your
own. The worst of them would have been escaped
if the facts had been disclosed to us before the
ruling was declared. A statute of New York, for-
bidding night work for women, was declared
arbitrary and void by a decision of the Court of
Appeals announced in 1907 (People *v*. Williams,
189 N. Y. 131). In 1915, with fuller knowledge
of the investigations of scientists and social
workers, a like statute was held by the same court
to be reasonable and valid (People *v*. Schweinler
Press, 214 N. Y. 395). "Courts know today"
(if I may borrow my own words) "that statutes
are to be viewed, not in isolation or *in vacuo*, as
pronouncements of abstract principles for the
guidance of an ideal community, but in the
setting and the framework of present-day condi-

tions as revealed by the labors of economists and students of the social sciences in our own country and abroad" (Cardozo, *The Nature of the Judicial Process*, p. 81).

Examples to point the meaning come flocking at the call. Again and again we are asked to nullify legislation as an undue encroachment upon the sphere of individual liberty. Encroachment to some extent there is by every command or prohibition. Liberty in the literal sense is impossible for anyone except the anarchist, and anarchy is not law, but its negation and destruction. What is undue in mandate or restraint cannot be known in advance of the event by a process of deduction from metaphysical principles of unvarying validity. It can be known only when there is knowledge of the mischief to be remedied, and knowledge of the mischief — to which, of course, must be added knowledge of the effectiveness of the remedy to counteract or cure the mischief — is knowledge of the facts. We do not turn to a body of esoteric legal doctrine, at least not invariably, to find the key to some novel problem of constitutional limitation, the bounds of permissible encroachment on liberty or property. We turn at times to physiology or embryology or chemistry or medicine — to a Jenner or a Pasteur or a Virchow or a Lister as freely and submissively as to a Blackstone or a Coke. Of course, even then we try to know our place and exhibit the humility that becomes the amateur. We do not assume to sit in judgment between conflicting schools of thought. Enough it is for us that the view embodied in a contested statute has at least respectable support — its sponsors, if perchance its critics — in the true abodes of science. Shall hours of labor be limited in one calling or another, for this group or for that? The physiologist as well as the sociologist must supply us with the body of knowledge appropriate to the problem to be solved. Such cases as People *v.* The Schweinler Press, (214 N. Y. 395), decided by the Court of Appeals of New York in 1915, and Muller *v.* Oregon, (208 U. S. 412), decided in 1908 by the Supreme Court of the United States, show the answer of the courts when the enlightening facts were put before them by workers in other fields. Shall compulsory vaccination be exacted of the children in the public shcools? Read the answer of the courts in Matter of Viemeister, (179 N. Y. 235), decided in 1904, and Jacobson *v.* Massachusetts, (197 U. S. 11), decided a year later. Only the other day my court had to deal with the propriety of the tuberculin test as applied to herds of cattle, the unfortunates who responded to the test being marked for quarantine or slaughter (People *v.* Teuscher, July, 1928, 248 N. Y. 454). A question of scientific fact is at the core of other problems, juridical in form, and yet intense, or so I hear, in their emotional appeal. What is a beverage, and when is it intoxicating? Let me not open ancient wounds by a reminder of the answer.

We look then to you, to the students of mind and body, for the nutriment of fact, solid if not liquid, that in many a trying hour will give vitality and vigor to the tissues of our law. Conspicuously is this true today in the administration of the law of crime. The law of crime has dramatic features which make it bulk large in the public mind, though of all the cases in my court the criminal appeals make up a small proportion, say eight or ten per cent. None the less, from the viewpoint of its social consequences the criminal law has an importance that is imperfectly reflected in statistical averages or the tables of accountants. The field is one in which the physician is asserting himself year by year with steadily expanding power. Among students of criminology there are now many who maintain that the whole business of sentencing criminals should be taken away from the judges and given over to the doctors. Courts, with their judges and juries, are to find the fact of guilt or innocence. The fact being ascertained, the physician is to take the prisoner in hand and say what shall be done with him. Governor Smith in his message to the Legislature of 1928 recommended that this reform be studied by the Crime Commission. "Because," he said, "of my belief that justice sometimes miscarries because those charged with determining guilt are often affected by the thought of the sentence to be imposed for a given crime, I would suggest that the Crime Commission give careful study and consideration to a fundamental change in the method of sentencing criminals. After guilt has been determined by legal process, instead of sentence being fixed by judges according to statute, I should like to see offenders who have been adjudged guilty detained by the state. They should then be carefully studied by a board of expert mental and physical specialists, who after careful study of all the elements entering each case would decide and fix the penalty for the crime. I realize the complexity of such a fundamental change. It probably requires even constitutional amendment. Therefore I recommend that your honorable bodies request the Crime

Commission to report to you, after due and careful study of the proposal, whether such a change is advisable and how it can be brought about. It appeals to me as a modern, humane, scientific way to deal with the criminal offender."

The reform thus proposed is no extemporized nostrum, no hasty innovation. It was recommended not many years ago by a committee of the Institute of Criminal Law and Criminology, of which the chairman was Victor P. Arnold, judge of the Juvenile Court of Chicago. This committee proposed *inter alia* "that in all cases of felony or misdemeanors punishable by a prison sentence the question of responsibility be not submitted to the jury, which will thus be called upon to determine only that the offense was committed by the defendant," and "that the disposition and treatment (including punishment) of all such misdemeanants and felons — *i.e.*, the sentence imposed, be based upon a study of the individual offender by properly qualified and impartial experts coöperating with the courts" (10 *Journal Criminal Law and Criminology*, p. 186; Glueck, *Mental Disorder and the Criminal Law*, p. 455). One of the most careful studies of the crime problem in recent years is that of Dr. S. Sheldon Glueck in his work on *Mental Disorder and the Criminal Law.* "If," he says (pp. 485, 486), "the socio-legal treatment of *all* criminals regardless of pathological condition, were being considered, it would seem that the simplest device would be to permit the law to convict or acquit as is done today, but to provide for *an administrative* instrumentality (perhaps a commission composed of psychiatrists, psychologists, sociologists, and others) to begin to function in case of convicted persons at the point where the law leaves off, to determine the appropriate socio-penal treatment adequate to the individual delinquent, as well as its duration." Developing this thought in an interesting essay, "A Rational Penal Code," published in the *Harvard Law Review*, (41 *Harvard Law Review* 453), he puts forward the view that the miniumum sentence should be fixed by law, but that the maximum in every instance should be left indefinite, to be determined for the individual prisoner by psychiatrists and physicians after a study of the individual case (cf. Gillin, *Criminology and Penology*, p. 153). Even now in some of the countries of continental Europe — in Switzerland, for example — a criminal whose mentality is low, though insanity is not suspected, is turned over for examination to psychiatrists in the service of the government, who make their recommendations to the court before sentence is pronounced.[1]

Not a little impetus has been given to these and like reforms by researches of bio-chemists into the operations of the ductless glands. If most of their conclusions are still in the stage of speculation or hypothesis, their writings have been useful, none the less, in awaking popular interest in the mentality of criminals, bringing home the need of study and the possibilities of a reformed penology to many who were blissfully unconscious of the existence of a problem. Our vices as well as our virtues have been imputed to bodily derangements till character has become identified with a chemical reaction. "The internal secretions," says an enthusiastic student of the endocrines (Berman, *The Glands Regulating Personality*, p. 22), "the internal secretions with their influence upon brain and nervous system, as well as every other part of the body-corporation, as essentially blood-circulating chemical

---

[1] (Cf. the recent statute of Massachusetts, l. 1927, c. 59, which calls for an examination by psychiatrists of any person indicted for a capital offense or any person indicted for another offense after an earlier conviction for a felony. Such a statute will do much to remove the reproach that has attached so long and so persistently to the testimony of experts; see 13 *Mass. Law Quarterly*, p. 38, *et seq.*, No. 6, August, 1828.)

substances, have been discovered the real governors and arbiters of instincts and dispositions, emotions and reactions, characters and temperaments, good and bad." A far cry is this from the voice of Socrates in the *Republic* of Plato: "My belief is, not that a good body will by its own excellence make the soul good; but, on the contrary, that a good soul will by *its* excellence render the body as perfect as it can be." The criminal of old was given copious draughts of exhortation and homily administered with solemn mien by reformers lay and cleric. The criminal of tomorrow will have fewer homilies and exhortations, but will have his doses of thyroxin or adrenalin till his being is transfigured. Good people sitting peacefully in their homes and reading fearsome tales of robbery and rapine, may take comfort in the thought that while the regeneration of character is in this process of "becoming," the body of the offender will be in the keeping of the law.

I have no thought in all this to express approval or disapproval of the project of withdrawing from the court the sentence-fixing power. One may see a wise reform there without acceptance of the creed that virtue and vice are not spiritual essences, but high-sounding synonyms for the hormones of the body. As to this last many of us, perhaps in our ignorance, will feel like echoing the words of Principal Jacks in his suggestive little book, *Constructive Citizenship*. "I think also," he says, "that while most of us are content to have our vices (but not our virtues) explained in this charitable manner by our neighbors, very few of us, and those the meanest, are in the habit of applying it to themselves. When we apply it to ourselves, a voice within seems to answer 'It is false.'" He is speaking, as it happens, of another and earlier precept of criminology, the precept that virtue and vice are the products solely of environment, but his words are as apposite to the notion that they are the products chiefly of the glands, though in each case it is true that repugnance must not be taken as amounting to disproof. All this, however, is beside the mark, at least for present purposes. Like the neophytes of other faiths, the discoverers of the new theory that virtue and vice are synonyms for spontaneous secretions may have overshot the mark, may have loaded a useful notion with more than it can bear. To prove that genius is accompanied by certain bodily changes or creations is not to prove that the bodily changes or reactions are identical with genius (cf. Bertrand Russell, *Philos-*

ophy, p. 218). This does not detract from the fullness of my belief that at a day not far remote the teachings of bio-chemists and behaviorists, of psychiatrists and penologists, will transform our whole system of punishment for crime. Vain is the attempt to forecast here and now the lines of the transfigured structure. We must keep a sharp lookout, or you will supplant us altogether. Do they not tell the fable of Hippocrates that he burned the library of the Temple of Health at Cnidos in order to enjoy a monopoly of knowledge? How it will work out, whether we shall sit beside you or above you, or even perhaps below you, I am not wise enough to say. The physician may be merely the ally of the judge in the business of admeasuring the sentence, or, as to that branch of the work, may even drive the judge away. Detention of the offender may retain in respect of certain crimes the qualities, or some of them, belonging to our present system of imprisonment, and for other crimes may acquire a quality less punitive and rigorous. But transformation there will be.

For the present system is stern often when it should be mild, and mild often when it should be stern, or so, at least, its critics urge. It is a survival of the time when punishment for crime was thought of as a substitute for private vengeance, with its sequel private war. The familiar phrase, the King's Peace, means this and nothing more, that for the peace separately maintained by duke or count or bishop, each in his own domain, there was to be substituted one general or uniform peace, the king's, establishing a single rule throughout the kingdom far and wide. You will find it all set forth by Sir Frederick Pollock in one of his fascinating essays with the fullness of example that is dear to antiquarians (Pollock, Oxford Lectures, *The King's Peace*, p. 64). We have put away the blood feud, the vendetta, the other forms of private war, but in the framing of our penal codes we have not forgotten the passions that had their outlet and release in pursuit and retribution. I do not say that it is wise to forget them altogether. The thirst for vengeance is a very real, even if it be a hideous, thing; and states may not ignore it till humanity has been raised to greater heights than any that have yet been scaled in all the long ages of struggle and ascent. Disregard such passions altogether, and the alternative may be the recrudescence of the duel or the feud. The vigilance committee and Judge Lynch may shove aside police and courts. Even if vengeance be forgotten and the social consequences alone considered, there are inhibitions in the threat of punishment that society cannot afford to withdraw from any capable of feeling them. "The presence of mechanism," says Dr. Glueck (*op. cit.,* p. 444), "does not mean that human beings have not some spark of capacity for consciously and creatively guiding their conduct in conformity with legal sanctions." Punishment is necessary, indeed, not only to deter the man who is a criminal at heart, who has felt the criminal impulse, who is on the brink of indecision, but also to deter others who in our existing social organization have never felt the criminal impulse and shrink from crime in horror. Most of us have such a scorn and loathing of robbery or forgery that the temptation to rob or forge is never within the range of choice; it is never a real alternative. There can be little doubt, however, that some of this repugnance is due to the ignominy that has been attached to these and like offenses through the sanctions of the criminal law. If the ignominy were withdrawn, the horror might be dimmed.

All this I have in mind, yet even so, the present system, in the view of many, is as irrational in its mercies as in its rigors, and in its rigors as in its mercies. The casual offender expiates

his offense in the company of defectives and re-
cidivists, and after devastating years is given
back an outcast to the society that made him.
The defective or recidivist, whose redemption is
hopeless, goes back after a like term, or one not
greatly different, to renew his life of crime, un-
able to escape it without escaping from himself.
Students of the mind and body are insisting, as
never before, that in much of our criminology
there is futility and waste. "It is foolish," says
one of them, "to build institutions for detaining
defectives for long periods as a punishment for a
condition for which they are not responsible, and
then discharge them without doing anything to
remove the cause of their trouble." "For a large
proportion of criminals," says another author,
"— the percentage has yet to be determined —
punishment for a period of time and then letting
him go free is like imprisoning a diphtheria-carrier
for a while and then permitting him to commingle
with his fellows and spread the germ of diph-
theria" (S. W. Bandler, *The Endocrines*, p. 266;
Berman, *The Glands Regulating Personality*, p. 310;
Schlapp and Smith, *The New Criminology*, p. 270).
A beginning of a change has been made in this
state by recent legislation, but with tests, in the
thought of many, too mechanical and absolute.

Not improbably the path of progress has been marked in an English statute which supplements the term of punishment in prison with another and elastic term of what is known as preventive detention in less rigorous surroundings, a camp in the Isle of Wight being set aside for that use (Gillin, *Criminology and Penology*, p. 412; Preventive of Crime Act, 8 Edw. 7 c. 59; Halsbury Laws of England, Title Crim. L., § 796).[1] Here or in some system not dissimilar may be found the needed adjustment between the penal and the remedial elements in our scheme of criminology.

Adjustment of some sort there must be if we are to fill the measure of our duty to our defective fellow beings. Run your eyes over the life history of a man sentenced to the chair. There, spread before you in all its inevitable sequence, is a story of the Rake's Progress more implacable than any that was ever painted by a Hogarth. The Correctional School, the Reformatory, Sing Sing or Dannemora, and then at last the chair.

[1] On the same lines a recent amendment of the Prison Law of New York permits the detention of mental defectives at the State Institution at Napanoch after sentence has expired (Prison Law, §§ 467, 470; Laws of 1927, chap. 426), but the term mental defectives as used in the statute (Mental Hygiene Law, § 136) embraces a narrower class than the same term is meant to embrace as it is used in this address. Very likely an extension of these provisions to prisoners of other types may be expected in the future.

The heavy hand of doom was on his head from the beginning. The sin, in truth, is ours — the sin of a penal system that leaves the victim to his fate when the course that he is going is written down so plainly in the files of the courts and the stigmata of mind and body. I do not mean to say that any rule of thumb is to be adopted in dealing with these problems. My experience as a judge in other fields of law has made me distrustful of rules of thumb generally. They are a lazy man's expedient for ridding himself of the trouble of thinking and deciding. Try hard as we will, the problems of punishment, like the problems of law generally, are in their essence unique. "We must spread the gospel," writes Professor Powell, "we must spread the gospel that there is no gospel that will save us from the pain of choosing at every step." Human nature, like human life, has complexities and diversities too many and too intricate to be compressed within a formula. I would not shut the door of hope on anyone, though classified in some statistical table as defective or recidivist, so long as scientific analysis and study of his mental and physical reactions after the state had taken him in hand held out the promise of redemption. Neither in punishment nor in any other form of judging shall we ever rid ourselves altogether of the heart-breaking burden of individual adjustment.

I do not say that either psychology or medicine or penology has yet arrived at such a stage as to make a revolution in our system of punishment advisable or possible. Here as in so many fields we shall have to feel our way, it may be, by slow advances, by almost insensible approaches. I have faith, none the less, that a century or less from now, our descendants will look back upon the penal system of today with the same surprise and horror that fill our own minds when we are told that only about a century ago one hundred and sixty crimes were visited under English law with the punishment of death, and that in 1801 a child of thirteen was hanged at Tyburn for the larceny of a spoon (4 Blackstone, Comm. 18; cf. however, 1 Stephen, *History of the Criminal Law of England* 470). Dark chapters are these in the history of law. We think of them with a shudder, and say to ourselves that we have risen to heights of mercy and of reason far removed from such enormities. The future may judge us less leniently than we choose to judge ourselves (cf. Jung, *Das Problem des Natürlichen Rechts*, p. 74). Perhaps the whole business of the retention of the death penalty will seem to the next generation, as it seems to many even now, an anachronism too discordant to be suffered, mocking with grim reproach all our clamorous professions of the sanctity of life. Perhaps some new Howard will make us see in our whole prison system a reproach as great, a blot as dark, as the Howard of English history made visible to the eyes of all in the prisons and pest houses of a century and a half ago. I am not sure how this will be. Sure, however, I am that whatever enlightenment shall come will make its way, not through the unaided labors of the men of my profession, the judges and the advocates, but through the combined labors of men of many callings, and most of all your own. How quickly a great change can come about will be seen if we contrast the penal justice applied to children a quarter-century ago with the treatment in these days of the juvenile delinquent by the judges of the Children's Courts. You will find it all set forth in a recent study of Juvenile Courts in the United States by Dr. Herbert H. Lou in the Social Study Series of the University of North Carolina. The methods, the humane and scientific methods, that have thus prevailed will spread to other fields. This is your work, I am persuaded, as much as it is ours. Your hands must hold the torch that will explore the dark mystery of crime — the mystery, even darker, of the criminal himself, in all the deep recesses of thought and will and body. Here is a common ground, a borderland between your labors and our own, where hope and faith and love can do their deathless work.

One takes a large order when one offers to reshape from its foundations a scheme of penal justice. Those of us whose course has even now been largely run, may wish to have before us a prospect less Utopian. Let me call attention, therefore, to two features of the law of crimes where the coöperation of your profession will be helpful even now without wreaking our energies upon reforms that will flower at some distant day. I think the men of your Academy might well emphasize the need for a restatement of our law of homicide, and in particular of the distinction between murder in its two degrees. I think they might well emphasize another subject — one that has grown a trifle stale, but never to be abandoned till it has been settled right — the definition of insanity when viewed as an excuse for crime.

The law of homicide, and in particular the distinction between murder in the first and second degrees, may seem at first blush to be something that involves the mere technique of criminal law, and so a matter not for you, but one to be dealt with by the lawyers. The reason why I mention it to you is because the anomalies of the present distinction can be developed with special clearness and authority by the psychiatrist or the alienist or the student of psychology.

Homicide under our statute is classified as murder and as manslaughter, and murder itself has two degrees, a first and a second. "The killing of a human being, unless it is excusable or justifiable, is murder in the first degree when committed from a deliberate and premeditated design to effect the death of the person killed, or of another," as well as in certain other situations which, for the purpose of my present inquiry, it is not important to consider (Penal Law, § 1044). "Such killing of a human being is murder in the second degree, when committed with a design to effect the death of the person killed or of another, but without deliberation and premeditation" (Penal Law, §1046). There, you see, is the distinction, and it is at least verbally clear. Both first and second degree murder (laying aside the exceptions which I thought it unnecessary to state) require an intent to kill, but in the one instance it is deliberate and premeditated intent, and in the other it is not. If there is no intent to kill whatever, the grade (subject to exceptions) is reduced to manslaughter. I have said that on the face of the statute the distinction is clear enough. The difficulty arises when we try to discover what is meant by the words deliberate and premeditated. A long series of decisions, beginning many years ago, has given to these words a meaning that differs to some extent from the one revealed upon the surface. To deliberate and premeditate within the meaning of the statute, one does not have to plan the murder days or hours or even minutes in advance, as where one lies in wait for one's enemy or places poison in his food or drink. The law does not say that any particular length of time must intervene between the volition and the act. The human brain, we are reminded (People *v.* Majone 91 N. Y. 211), acts at times with extraordinary celerity. All that the statute requires is that the act must not be the result of immediate or spontaneous impulse. "If there is hesitation or doubt to be overcome, a choice made as the result of thought, however short the struggle between the intention and the act," there is such deliberation and premeditation as will expose the offender to the punishment of death (People *v.* Leighton, 88 N. Y. 117). Thus in a case decided in 1886

(People *v.* Beckwith, 103 N. Y. 360), the defendant ejected a trespasser; a fight ensued; the defendant stabbed the trespasser and flung him to the ground; having done this, he seized an ax and clove the victim's head. The interval between the knife blow and the falling ax was long enough to sustain the verdict that sent the murderer to his death. One may say indeed in a rough way that an intent to kill is always deliberate and premeditated within the meaning of the law unless the mind is so blinded by pain or rage as to make the act little more than an automatic or spontaneous reaction to the environment — not strictly automatic or spontaneous, for there could then be no intent, and yet a near approach thereto. The behaviorists would say, I suppose, that what had happened was a conditioned reflex, a learned, as opposed to an unlearned, response (Watson, *Behaviorism*, p. 103, and cf. B. Russell, *Philosophy*, p. 21). Courts in other states (*e.g.*, Massachusetts) lay down the same rule or rules not greatly different.

I think the distinction is much too vague to be continued in our law. There can be no intent unless there is a choice, yet by the hypothesis, the choice without more is enough to justify the inference that the intent was deliberate and premeditated. The presence of a sudden impulse is said to mark the dividing line, but how can an impulse be anything but sudden when the time for its formation is measured by the lapse of seconds? Yet the decisions are to the effect that seconds may be enough. What is meant, as I understand it, is that the impulse must be the product of an emotion or passion so swift and overmastering as to sweep the mind from its moorings. A metaphor, however, is, to say the least, a shifting test whereby to measure degrees of guilt that mean the difference between life and death. I think the students of the mind should make it clear to the lawmakers that the statute is framed along the lines of a defective and unreal psychology. If intent is deliberate and premeditated whenever there is choice, then in truth it is always deliberate and premeditated, since choice is involved in the hypothesis of the intent. What we have is merely a privilege offered to the jury to find the lesser degree when the suddenness of the intent, the vehemence of the passion, seems to call irresistibly for the exercise of mercy. I have no objection to giving them this dispensing power, but it should be given to them directly and not in a mystifying cloud of words. The present distinction is so obscure that no jury hearing it for the first time can fairly be expected to assimilate and understand it. I am not at all sure that I understand it myself after trying to apply it for many years and after diligent study of what has been written in the books. Upon the basis of this fine distinction with its obscure and mystifying psychology, scores of men have gone to their death. I think it is time for you who speak with authority as to the life of the mind to say whether the distinction has such substance and soundness that it should be permitted to survive. Some appropriate committee there should be in the bar associations, on the one hand, and this Academy, on the other (if none exists already), whereby the resources of the two professions can be pooled in matters such as these where society has so much to gain from coöperative endeavor.

I have spoken of another branch of the law of homicide, the law defining and governing mental irresponsibility. In strictness, this is not a branch of the law of homicide alone, since the same definition applies to other crimes as well, yet it is in connection with homicide that the question commonly arises. In the early stages of our law, way back in mediæval times, insanity was never a defense for crime. The insane killer, like the man who killed in self-defense, might seek a pardon from the king, and would often get one. He had no defense at law. Gradually there came in the law itself a mitigation of this rigor. A defense of insanity was allowed, but only within the narrowest limits. This was what has become known as the wild-beast stage of the defense. The killer was not excused unless he had so lost his mind as to be no more capable of understanding than if he were merely a wild beast. Then the limits of the defense were expanded, but still slowly and narrowly. The killer was excused if the disease of the mind was such that he was incapable of appreciating the difference between right and wrong. At first this meant, not the right and wrong of the particular case, but right and wrong generally or in the abstract, the difference, as it was sometimes said, between good and evil. Later the rule was modified in favor of the prisoner so that capacity to distinguish between right and wrong generally would not charge with responsibility if there was not capacity to understand the difference in relation to the particular act, the subject of the crime. The rule governing the subject was crystallized in England in 1843 by the answer made by the House of Lords to questions submitted by the judges in the famous case of McNaghten, who was tried for the murder of one Drummond, the secretary of Sir Robert Peel. The answer was in effect that "the jurors ought to be told in all cases that every man is to be presumed to be sane, and to possess a sufficient degree of reason to be responsible for his crimes, until the contrary be proved to their satisfaction; and that to establish a defense on the ground of insanity it must be clearly proved that, at the time of committing the act, the accused was laboring under such a defect of reason, from disease of the mind, as not to know the nature and quality of the act he was doing, or, if he did know it, that he did not know he was doing what was wrong" (McNaghten's Case, 10 Cl. & F. 200).

The test established by McNaghten's Case has been incorporated into the law of New York by the mandate of the statute. Penal Law, § 34, provides: "A person is not excused from criminal liability as an idiot, imbecile, lunatic or insane person, except upon proof that at the time of the commission of the alleged criminal act he was laboring under such a defect of reason as either (1) not to know the nature and quality of the act he was doing; (2) not to know the act was wrong." It matters not that some uncontrollable impulse, the product of mental disease, may have

driven the defendant to the commission of the
murderous act. The law knows nothing of such
excuses (Flanagan *v.* People, 52 N. Y. 467; People
v. Carpenter, 102 N. Y. 238; People *v.* Taylor,
138 N. Y. 398). Again the statute is explicit:
"A morbid propensity to commit prohibited
acts, existing in the mind of a person who is not
shown to have been incapable of knowing the
wrongfulness of such acts, forms no defense to a
prosecution therefor" (Penal Law, § 34). If the
offender knew the nature and quality of the act
and knew it to be wrong, he must answer for it
with his life, if death is the penalty that would
be paid by the sane. Of course, there is an am-
biguity in all this which will not have escaped
your quick discernment. What is meant by
knowledge that the act is wrong? Is it enough
that there was knowledge that the act was wrong
in the sense that it was prohibited by law, or
must there be knowledge also that it was mor-
ally wrong? Curiously enough, this question did
not arise in New York till 1915. One Schmidt,
a priest, was charged with the murder of a wo-
man with whom he had been intimate. Upon the
trial his defense was insanity. He said he had
heard the voice of God calling upon him by day
and night to sacrifice and slay. He yielded to the

call in the belief that slaughter was a moral duty. The trial judge held that this belief was no defense if he knew the nature of the act and knew it to be wrong in the sense of being prohibited by law. On appeal this ruling was reversed (People *v.* Schmidt, 216 N. Y. 324). We held that the word "wrong" in the statutory definition had reference in such circumstances to the moral quality of the act, and not merely to the legal prohibition. Any other reading would charge a mother with the crime of murder if she were to slay a dearly loved child in the belief that a divine command had summoned to the gruesome act. Let me say by way of parenthesis that Schmidt did not profit by the error in the charge, since he admitted under oath that the whole defense of insanity was an imposture and a sham.

Physicians time and again rail at the courts for applying a test of mental responsibility so narrow and inadequate. There is no good in railing at us. You should rail at the legislature. The judges have no option in the matter. They are bound, hand and foot, by the shackles of a statute. Everyone concedes that the present definition of insanity has little relation to the truths of mental life. There are times, of course, when a killing has occurred without knowledge by the killer of the nature of the act. A classic instance is the case of Mary Lamb, the sister of Charles Lamb, who killed her mother in delirium. There are times when there is no knowledge that the act is wrong, as when a mother offers up her child as a sacrifice to God. But after all, these are rare instances of the workings of a mind deranged. They exclude many instances of the commission of an act under the compulsion of disease, the countless instances for example, of crime by paranoiacs under the impulse of a fixed idea. I am not unmindful of the difficulty of framing a definition of insanity that will not be so broad as to open wide the door to evasion and imposture. Conceivably the law will have to say that the risk is too great, that the insane must answer with their lives, lest under cover of their privilege the impostor shall escape. Conceivably the twilight zone between sanity and insanity is so broad and so vague as to bid defiance to exact description. I do not know, though I am reluctant to concede that science is so impotent. Attempts at formulation of a governing principle or standard have been none too encouraging (Glueck, *op. cit.*, pp. 452, 459), but betterment is attainable, though it be something less than perfection. Many states — Massachusetts, for example, and Alabama and Pennsyl-

vania and Virginia and Vermont — recognize the
fact that insanity may find expression in an irre-
sistible impulse, yet I am not aware that the
administration of their criminal law has suffered
as a consequence (see, *e.g.*, Commonwealth *v.*
Cooper, 219 Mass. 1; Parsons *v.* State, 81 Ala.
577; Commonwealth *v.* DeMarzo, 223 Pa. St.
573; State *v.* Dejarnette, 75 Va. 867; Doherty *v.*
State, 73 Vt. 380). Much of the danger might
be obviated if the issue of insanity were triable
by a specially constituted tribunal rather than
the usual jury. Of this at least I am persuaded:
the medical profession of the state, the students
of the life of the mind in health and in disease,
should combine with students of the law in a
scientific and deliberate effort to frame a definition, and a system of administration, that will
combine efficiency with truth. If insanity is not
to be a defense, let us say so frankly and even
brutally, but let us not mock ourselves with
a definition that palters with reality. Such a
method is neither good morals nor good science
nor good law. I know it is often said, and
very likely with technical correctness, (see, *e.g.*,
Oppenheimer, *Criminal Responsibility of Luna-
tics*, p. 247; Stephen, *Digest of Criminal Law*,
Art. 29; Glueck, *op. cit.*, p. 43), that the stat-

ute ought not to be viewed as defining insanity. What it does, and all that it does is to state the forms or phases of insanity that will bring immunity from punishment. All this may be true, yet it is hard to read the statute without feeling that by implication and suggestion it offers something more. It keeps the word of promise to the ear and breaks it to the hope. Let us try to improve its science and at the very least its candor. Here is another field for the coöperative endeavor of medicine and law.

Every now and then there crops up in popular journals a discussion of the problem of euthanasia. The query is propounded whether the privilege should be accorded to a physician of putting a patient painlessly out of the world when there is incurable disease, agonizing suffering, and a request by the sufferer for merciful release. No such privilege is known to our law, which shrinks from any abbreviation of the span of life, shaping its policy in that regard partly under the dominance of the precepts of religion and partly in the fear of error or abuse. Just as a life may not be shortened, so its value must be held as equal to that of any other, the mightiest or the lowliest. The mother will have the preference over an infant yet unborn, but from the moment of birth onward, human-kind, as the law views it, is a society of equals. I am sure that thoughts of this order must rise sometimes to your minds when you move along the wards of hospitals and see the forms of men and women — the ugly and the beautiful, the wise and the foolish, the young and the old, the gay and the wretched — outstretched before you in the great democracy of suffering. You may find it of some interest to be told that the law has had to struggle with these problems and to know how it has resolved them. There are two classic cases — the case of the U. S. *v*. Holmes, reported in 1 Wallace, Jr., 1; Federal cases No. 15,383, a trial in the United States Circuit Court for the Eastern District of Pennsylvania, and the case of the Queen *v*. Dudley, reported in L. R. 14 Q. B. D. 273, a trial in the Court of Queen's Bench of England. The Holmes case has recently been revived with a full statement of the testimony, the arguments of counsel, and the charge of the court, in a book by Frederick C. Hicks, to which he has given the title *Human Jettison*. Any of you who care to read it will find a human document of absorbing interest. Holmes was a seaman on a ship, the *William Brown*, which set sail from Liverpool for Philadelphia in 1841 with eighty-two souls abroad, seventeen officers and crew, and sixty-five passengers. Thirty-seven days out the ship struck an iceberg and sank. Two boats were lowered. One, the jolly, as it was called, bore the captain, two officers, six members of the crew, and one passenger. Six days later, just as the rations had given out, she was picked up and those aboard her saved. The other boat, styled the long one, in the charge of the first mate, had forty-two aboard, of whom thirty-three were passengers, the others crew. The long boat was long only by comparison with the other. She was overweighted with her human burden — men, women, and children packed so close together in a boat already leaking that they could hardly move a limb. A squall came up the next day, and imminent was the danger that the boat would founder. The mate gave the order to jettison a portion of the human freight. Holmes and another carried out the mandate. Fourteen men were seized and, amid their protests and entreaties, were thrown over the side. Two women also were lost, but there is reason to believe that they jumped overboard of their own will, made desperate at the sight of the sacrifice of a brother. For the most part, however, the victims were the men. The boat, relieved of this burden, rode the waves in safety. The following morning a sail was sighted. Quilts and blankets were waved and hoisted. There was an answer to the signal. The ship came up and the remnant on the boat were saved.

When the story of the sacrifice of sixteen souls became known to the world, there were many who drew back revolted and said that it was murder. The mate and most of the seamen disappeared when there was talk of an arrest. Holmes came to Philadelphia and was charged with homicide on the high seas, a crime under the federal law. The grand jury refused to indict for murder, but did indict for manslaughter. For this he was tried and convicted. He was sentenced to imprisonment for six months, having already served nine months before his conviction, and also to a fine, which, however, was afterward remitted. I think there is little, if any, doubt that he had acted in good faith, believing that all would be lost unless there was a sacrifice of some. His good faith did not purge him of the guilt of crime, though it called for mercy in the sentence. Where two or more are overtaken by a common disaster, there is no right on the part of one to save the lives of some by the killing of another. There is no rule of human jettison.

Men there will often be who when told that
their going will be the salvation of the remnant,
will choose the nobler part and make the plunge
into the waters. In that supreme moment the
darkness for them will be illumined by the
thought that those behind will ride to safety. If
none of such mold are found aboard the boat, or
too few to save the others, the human freight
must be left to meet the chances of the waters.
Who shall choose in such an hour between the
victims and the saved? Who shall know when
masts and sails of rescue may emerge out of the
fog?

A score of years later a case not dissimilar was
brought before an English court. Three men and
a boy were adrift in a small boat. Two of the men,
Dudley and Stephens, made desperate by hun-
ger, killed the boy and ate his flesh. Four days
later they were picked up by a passing vessel,
and, reaching England, were tried for murder.
They were tried before an accomplished judge,
Lord Coleridge, Chief Justice of the Queen's
Bench. The jury returned a verdict of guilty,
but the sentence of death was commuted to one
of imprisonment for a term of months. The law
falters and averts her face and sheathes her own
sword when pronouncing judgment upon crea-

tures of flesh and blood thus goaded by the Furies.

One thing medicine has already done for jurisprudence, and that a thing so important as to exact a word of mention in even the briefest statement of the relations between the two. For many years medicine has been laying stress upon the value of institutes of mere research. You will find a sketch of their history in Dr. Abraham Flexner's *Study of Medical Education*. The law has been a little slower in the acceptance of such methods and ideals, yet at last it has seen the light. I cannot doubt that your example has done much to open our eyes and sharpen our perceptions. Research is now the cry in the schools of law at Harvard, Yale, Columbia, Michigan, and elsewhere. They are seeking to train the practitioner who some day may develop, or, shall I say, descend, into a judge, but they are seeking to do more. They are seeking to train the scholars — the jurists in the true sense of that much-abused term — who will lead the vanguard of the march. Only the other day, Johns Hopkins University, which has done so much already to stimulate the growth of medicine, announced the formation of an Institute of Jurisprudence, devoted to research and nothing else. A group of scholars has been brought together, who at the beginning will have no pupils other than themselves. They have come together to meditate, to confer, to collate, to explore. They will study the law functionally, asking themselves not merely whether this or that rule has come down to us from mediæval days, but whether this rule or that one is adapted to the present needs of life. So the spirit of disinterested inquiry, which has long inspired the students of the physical sciences, is spreading, we may justly believe, to the social sciences as well. I do not mean to convey the thought that the law which is mere innovation, a forced plant, so to speak, without roots in habit or custom or popular conviction, is to be looked to with great hopefulness as a curative or helpful force. What I fear and would avoid is the law that maintains a noxious life when the soil of habit and custom and conviction and utility has been washed away beneath it. I have no delusions as to the futility of mere extempore decretals. Even when changes are made, it is best at the beginning to mark out the general lines of tendency and direction, leaving details to be developed by the system of trial and error which is of the essence of the judicial process. "It is a peculiar virtue of our system of law" — the words are those of one of the great judges of our day — "that the process of inclusion and exclusion, so often employed in developing a rule, is not allowed to end with its enunciation, and that an expression in an opinion yields later to the impact of facts unforeseen" (Brandeis, J., dissenting, in Jaybird Mining Co. *v*. Weir, 271 U. S. 609). We must not sacrifice this quality of resilient adaptability which persists while there is softness and suppleness in the bones of legal doctrine. I do not say that it is an easy matter to find a just mean between timidity and boldness, or, to put it from another aspect, between literature and dogma. In case of doubt I have a leaning, which is not always shared by others, toward the impressionism that suggests and illumines without defining and imprisoning. The prevailing tendency is perhaps the other way, and the majority may be right. They hold the mysticism of the impressionist to be incompatible with the dignity of science. I am satisfied that this is so when science has so experimented as to have the right to be certain of its ground. What I fear is a pseudo-science which has assurance without conviction. Very likely in this mental attitude I am exemplifying what has been described by a learned author as "the invertebrate habit of mind which thinks it is impartial merely because it is undecided, and regards the judicial attitude as that which refrains from judging" (Dr. Figgis, Introduction to Lord Acton's *The History of Freedom and Other Essays*). When the seas are so boisterous and their perils so insidious, one creeps from cape to cape.

The law, like medicine, has its record of blunders and blindnesses and superstitions and even cruelties. Like medicine, however, it has never lacked the impulse of a great hope, the vision of a great ideal. Sometimes secreted in ancient forms and ceremonies one finds the inner life and meaning of an institution revealed in all its essence. I felt this not long ago while reading the form of oath administered even now in all its ancient beauty to the grand jurors of the county. You will find it in the Code of Criminal Procedure, but one not greatly different is in use by our English brethren in their home across the seas, and Sir Frederick Pollock has traced it back, in germ at least, to the days of the Saxon kings. In fitness and beauty and impressiveness it rivals the great oath that men associate even today with the name and genius of Hippocrates. Here is its form as it has endured through all the changing centuries: "You shall diligently inquire, and true presentment make, of all such matters and things as shall be given you in charge; the counsel of the people of this state, your fellows' and your own you shall keep secret; you shall present no person from envy, hatred and malice; nor shall you leave any one unpresented through fear, favor, affection or reward, or hope thereof; but you shall present all things truly as they come to your knowledge, according to the best of your understanding. So help you God!"

Like the tones of a mighty bell, these echoing notes of adjuration bring back our straying thoughts to sanctity and service. I cannot listen to them without a thrill. Here, I say to myself, here indeed, secreted in this solemn formula, is the true spirit of the law which knows no fear nor favor. Not all her ministers have been true to the ideal which she has held aloft for them to follow. But here, imperishably preserved amid the grime and dust of centuries, the word has been proclaimed, to steady us when we seem to falter, to strengthen us when we seem to weaken, to tell us that with all the failings and backslidings, with all the fears and all the prejudice, the spirit is still pure.

And so it still is for the great profession that is mine, as still it is for yours, which year by year renews in conduct and in speech the pledge and promise of Hippocrates.

I thank you for the privilege that has been given me of bringing the two together in this hall of your Academy.

Comment of Appreciation

No member of either profession — Medicine or Law — could have heard or can read Chief Judge Cardozo's address before the New York Academy of Medicine without being profoundly impressed by its message. It is an inspiring summons to the service of the community, and the answer of both professions cannot be doubtful. Their truest and greatest glory lies in the constant and vivifying spirit of public service which animates their members, and the permanent value of the present address arises from its lucid delineation of a field of labor in which the collaboration of the two professions seems to have become imperative.

With all the magic of style, the scholarly author at the outset of his review carries our minds back to pagan days and pagan gods. The custom which he recalls, attributed to primitive men, of classifying medicine and law as functions of both king and priest was dictated by a natural and common instinct. The two greatest and deepest interests of man on earth have ever been health and justice, and both were for ages instinctively coupled as equally the attributes and gifts of divinity. Amongst the ancients, the preference was perhaps given to medicine, as evidenced by Cicero's familiar saying *Homines ad deos nulla re propius accedunt quam salutem hominibus dando.* In nothing do men more nearly approach the gods than in giving health to men.

Judge Cardozo analyzes some of the duties and tasks which are facing both professions and calling for collaboration, study, elucidation and accurate definition; and he particularly emphasizes the practical problems arising from present methods in the administration of the criminal law. He points out, as illustrations, the urgent need of a really scientific definition of the crime of murder as well as a like definition of insanity, or rather the degree of mental disease that should be deemed an excuse for crime, or, stated in a different way, that should render it cruel, futile and uncivilized to inflict punishment on the mentally irresponsible when it cannot serve as a deterrent to others under like conditions.

In defining such legal terms as "intent" and "insanity," and fixing their essential content when employed in our penal laws, it can no longer be rational to adhere to rigid legalistic formulae or data gathered only from the character and extent of crime or the practical administration or enforcement of the criminal law, whilst disregarding the facts, the rules and the laws that are being constantly discovered by the students of the life of the mind in health and in disease. Competent experts and students of the operations and characteristics of the mind are pre-eminently to be found in the ranks of the medical profession; and the path of law enforcement must be too often haphazard and in darkness if the work of these experts be disregarded. Enlightenment must come from the results of their labors in the field of the newly developing sciences of psychology and psychiatry.

The legal task of accurate definition in penal law now requires acquaintance with the practical experience, the discoveries and the accomplishments of physicians, and their conceptions as to what is termed moral responsibility. Data in respect of these important terms gathered and analyzed by competent psychologists and psychiatrists would, undoubtedly, lead to a fundamental and far-reaching readjustment of the penal and remedial elements in the administration of our criminal law.

The field to which Judge Cardozo, the philosopher, calls the attention of both professions is very broad and will constantly present new and complex problems. For example, shall there be a differentiation between the process of ascertaining and determining guilt and the process of fixing the treatment or punishment of the guilty? Is adequate punishment an objective to be determined solely by fixed and unbending rules having no relation to individual idiosyncracies, or to the special facts in any particular case? Shall efforts to reclaim be guided by experts in the ever-varying phases, tendencies, qualities and diseases of the human mind as found in offenders against the law? The importance and gravity of these problems must be obvious to all who reflect upon the rigid, antiquated and unsatisfactory fashion in which criminals, young and old, are now being dealt with. All the advocates of the scientific treatment of criminals after they have been found guilty by the courts of justice are not sentimentalists or inclined to coddle the criminal; they are not seeking to abolish punishment; but rather, as has been well said, to make it effective by basing it upon intelligent investigation and ascertained fact and humane principles, to the end that, so modified, punishment will really begin successfully to function as a cure for crime, instead of tending, as it now too often does, to make it inveterate. Indeed, the future security of our civilization, the welfare and happiness of those who follow us, may depend in great measure upon intelligent and competent co-operation and collaboration between the two professions in solving this vital and eternal problem.

The Chief Judge warns us that he has no thought to express approval or disapproval of the project of withdrawing from the court the sentence-fixing power, though that momentous step, he recognizes, should only be taken, if at all, after much more research and study. The subject is yet too speculative. His admonition, however, is that, although he may be confident that there will be some form of transformation in the treatment of the two-fold problem of the enforcement of the law and protection of society on the one hand and the punishment and reclamation or reform of the offender on the other hand, nevertheless the change must be by slow and cautious advances and by almost insensible approaches. He then finely and truly adds that in the course of these advances and approaches the two professions will find a common ground or borderland in which the medical profession must now lead the way and "hold the torch that will explore the dark mystery of crime — the mystery, even darker, of the criminal himself, in all the deep recesses of thought and will and body."

In both professions, Judge Cardozo's address will truly inspire the impulse of a great hope, the vision of a great ideal, to which he nobly appeals. His elevated language must be a gospel of service and aspiration for lawyer and physician alike.

Shortly after the delivery of Judge Cardozo's address before the Academy of Medicine, the Association of the Bar of the City of New York appointed a special committee and charged it with the duty of co-operating with the Academy of Medicine and considering and making recommendations concerning his suggestions. A similar committee was appointed by the Academy of Medicine, which was likewise charged reciprocally with the duty of co-operating with the committee of the Association of the Bar. The collaboration of these two committees should ensure that the views outlined in Judge Cardozo's address will be thoroughly investigated and studied by groups of competent experts representing the legal and medical professions. In thus collaborating, the two professions will undoubtedly promote the scientific and beneficent development of medico-legal jurisprudence.

WILLIAM D. GUTHRIE
Ex-President Association of the Bar
of the City of New York

SAMUEL W. LAMBERT, M.D.
Ex-President of the New York
Academy of Medicine

www.ingramcontent.com/pod-product-compliance
Lightning Source LLC
Chambersburg PA
CBHW021433180326
41458CB00001B/256